AF426431

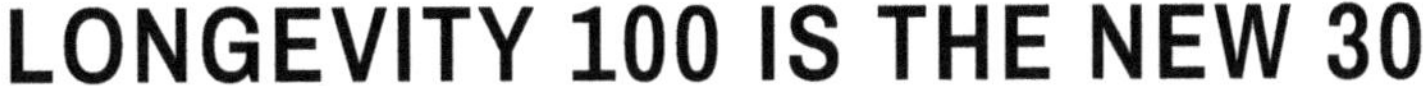
LONGEVITY 100 IS THE NEW 30

LONGEVITY 100 IS THE NEW 30

CINDY MARTIN NAGEL

This book is dedicated to anybody who believes they have the potential to live a long life. Look at my mother, who is still alive and is ninety-six, almost ninety-seven years old. My father lived up to ninety-four. Take note and follow the steps mentioned in the book; you can live as long as they and my other family members did.

My mother, a devoted Christian and God-fearing person., is still living her best life by taking care of herself and would like to see more years to come with the help of God

Pray a lot and eat well.

Table of Contents

Background: Family members who lived over 95 years old
Chapter 1: Introduction on Longevity
Chapter 2: Nutrient and diet
 Chapter 3:Exercise and Longevity
Chapter 4: Mental and emotional well-being
Chapter 5: Social Relationships
Chapter 6: Sleep and Restoration
Chapter 7: Lifelong Learning and Cognitive Health
Chapter 8: Preventive healthcare and regular checkups
Chapter 9: The Role of Technology and Innovation in Ageing
Chapter 10: Philosophy and Spirituality finding purpose in later life
Conclusion

Family Background

B<u>ackground of my family's history on how they lived over 90 years</u>
 My mother Muriel Martin Donatien is 97 years and is still alive and healthy. She has no health issues except for some pain in her knees.

She was born in Trinidad and Tobago which is located in the west indies. At the age of 34, she migrated to the United States of America.

From there, she worked hard and continued to eat properly and reading her bible was always a part of her everyday life. She has never been hospitalized for a day in her life only to have her 2 children which includes me and my older sister.

My mother does not believe in taking medication because she always says that tablets would do harm to your body than good. In addition, it is very important for her to eat healthy and exercise.

She loves to read and reading the health book inspired her to continue eating healthy and living a longer life.

Right before breakfast, my mother would do a 15-minute exercise in her room.

Her breakfast would consist of whole wheat bread with some butter. For fruits, she would either have strawberries, blueberries, grapes, or watermelon. She loves oatmeal and would add some cinnamon which would give it some flavor. Spices is also good for arthritis.

In her lunch hour, she would eat some brown rice with kale and avocados. Alongside her lunch, she would have cucumbers, boiled carrots, and a salad. For her drink, she would either water or a small glass of orange just. Drinking 8 glasses a water a day is necessary for her as it keeps her skin nice and smooth.

Diner was always light. It includes an apple, orange and a slice of whole grain bread with some fruit juice.

Her motto is, never stress too much about anything because God would handle it in his own time. Stress can also take a toll on your body, and in turn cause illnesses which can lead to death. Sleeping was a plus for her and she went to be 8pm every night.

During her upbringing, her parents believed in eating healthily. Which also means less visits to the doctor. So, they ate a lot of vegetables and fruits. Sweets and junk food were never included in their everyday diet.

My mother is still around to see up to her 4th generation.

My father Bernard Donatien lived up to 94 years old before he passed away in 2016. He suffered from high blood pressure because his parents had high blood pressure as well. My mother would encourage him to eat less salt and eat a lot of fresh fruits and vegetables.

He used to walk every day around the park for about 20 minutes. My mother never encourages him to take his blood pressure medication that the doctor prescribed him. She used to give him garlic with his meals with some water. This helped him a lot along with his walks everyday to maintain his blood pressure. Sleep is also important and he used to go to bed by 9pm every night,

My cousin Virginia Laura Boyce lived up to 104 years of age until she passed away in August of 2024.

Virgina Laura Boyce also came from Trinidad and Tobago and migrated to the United States in 1966.

She worked very hard during her time of life and maintained her health by eating fruits and vegetables and drinking a lot of water until she passed away.

My cousin Sue also lived up to 92 years of age and just passed away in September of 2024. She also maintained her health by eating healthy. Fruits and vegetables and drinking a lot of water was also important to her

Ena Boyce, my cousin (Virginia Laura Boyce's sister) lived up to 100 years of age until she passed away not too long ago. Ena also migrated from Trinidad and worked a lot in her garden. She grew her own fruits and vegetables. This was a way she maintained her health by eating from her garden. No preservatives or no chemicals. It was natural straight from her garden.

My mother-in-law lived up to 92 years of age until she died February of 2023. She migrated from Germany in 1964. I stayed with her for a while and her meals were small. Her breakfast consisted of a cup of coffee with no milk, blended grains and a slice of brown toast.

Lunch would be chicken or beef with a big salad.

Dinner was fruit and some fruit juice.

Moving forward, in this book, I would indicate ways on how to live long and stay healthy like my family members did.

CHAPTER 1

Introduction on Longevity

Longevity is a goal of striving for the maximum potential age which can be reached by practicing healthy behaviors and activities. In addition to longevity, it includes quality of life so you can live longer. Longevity has increased dramatically since 1900.

People who maintained five healthy lifestyle factors lived more than a decade longer than those who didn't maintain their health. (Here are the 5 factors that would help you live longer.

1. Healthy: Eat a balanced diet with many fruits and vegetables, whole grains, nuts, and healthy fats. Cut down on low-processed meats, sugary beverages, and sodium.
2. Exercise regularly: It is important to exercise 3 to 5 hours a week. It will prevent diseases and encourage overall well-being.
3. Do not smoke: If you stop smoking, it will lower the risk of heart disease, cancer, and other health issues.
4.) Drink less: You can drink but in moderation. Women can drink one glass per day, whereas men can have two glasses per day.
5. Keep your weight in check: Your body mass index (BM) should be 18.5 and 24.9

If you follow these steps and eat everything in moderation, you will be on your way to a long, healthier life.

There are nine foods that can help you live a longer life. What you eat is what you are and can make a significant change to your life. Your life span can be determined by genetics. Genes may only be 20% of how long you live.

-Berries

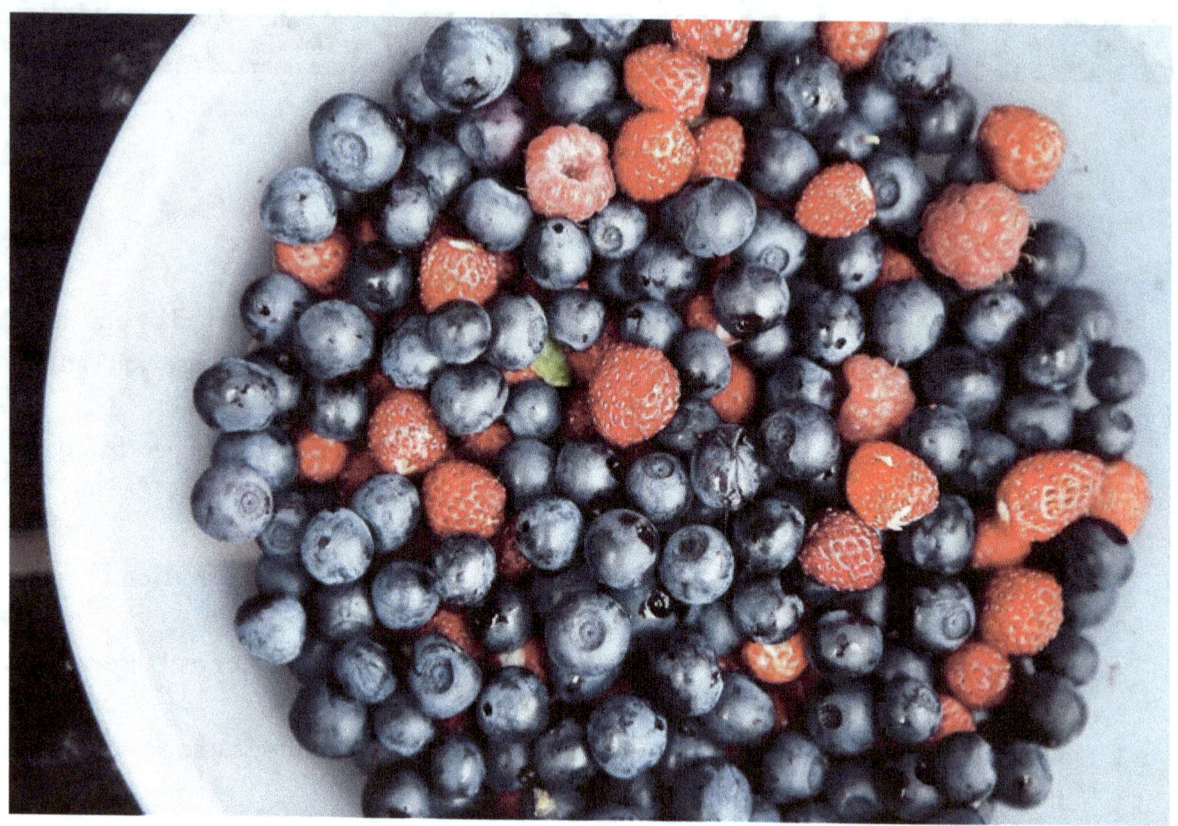

Berries have long been studied for health benefits ranging from reducing the risk of <u>cardiovascular disease</u> to <u>protection against cancer</u> and <u>lower levels of inflammation</u>

What's even more intriguing about berries is their potential effect on brain health.

"Whether you favor strawberries, raspberries, blueberries, or blackberries, they all offer health-protective vitamins, minerals, antioxidants and fiber. The antioxidant content of blueberries, raspberries, and blackberries also ranks among the highest of all fruits and enables them to combat free radicals that can cause damage to your cells, as well as inflammation, says Stark.

In many regions, fresh berries are only available (or affordable) for a few short months of the year, but frozen berries are just as nutritious as they are picked at their peak ripeness. Enjoy them straight out of the container as a snack; on your yogurt or oatmeal; in a salad or smoothie; or made into a salsa for fish or poultry.

-Kale

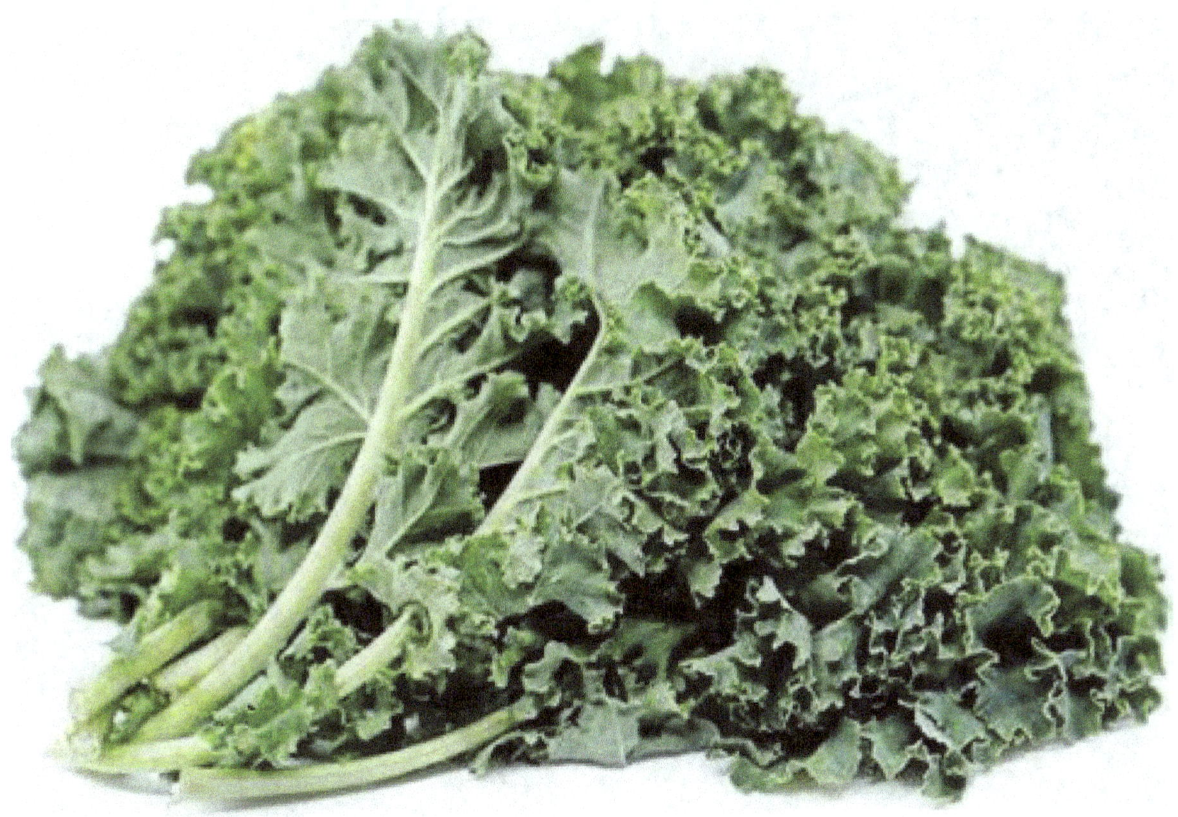

Kale is based on lutein and zeaxanthin. It also increases skin elasticity, hydration, and fat under the skin. However, it plays a part in making the skin stay youthful. It also protects the skin from harmful wavelengths called lutein. Sunscreen is never used because it is not very good at protecting the skin against the sun. Avocado is also full of lutein and should be eaten every day.

-Dark Chocolate

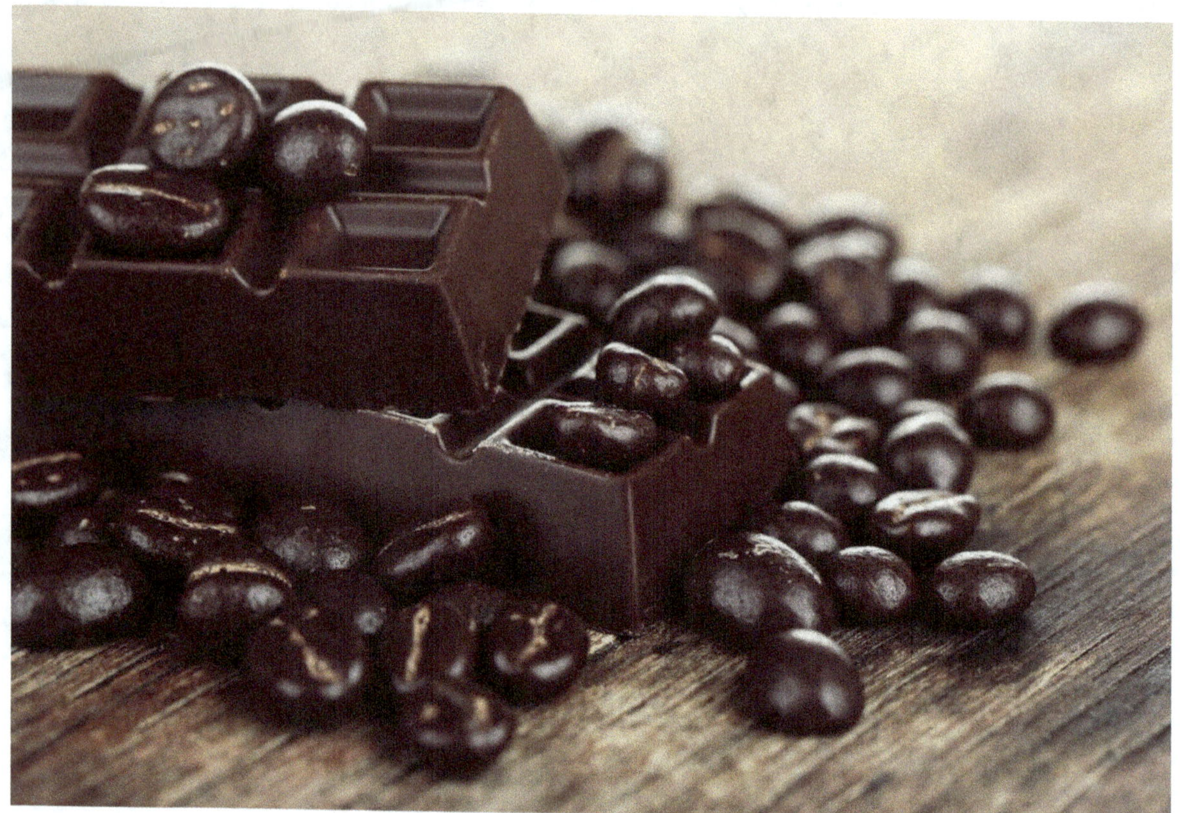

Dark Chocolate is an anti-aging benefit. What makes up dark chocolate, is cocoa beans and it is loaded with antioxidants that can decrease inflammation from UV exposure. It has a function that can increase function that can increase circulation and help the skin to better retain moisture. This keeps the skin looking healthy and fresh. Magnesium is also linked to dark chocolate, which keeps stress levels low and improves sleep; not getting enough sleep increases the aging process.

Dark chocolate contains a lot of sugar and can cause havoc to the skin, but you can eat it in moderation.

-Spices

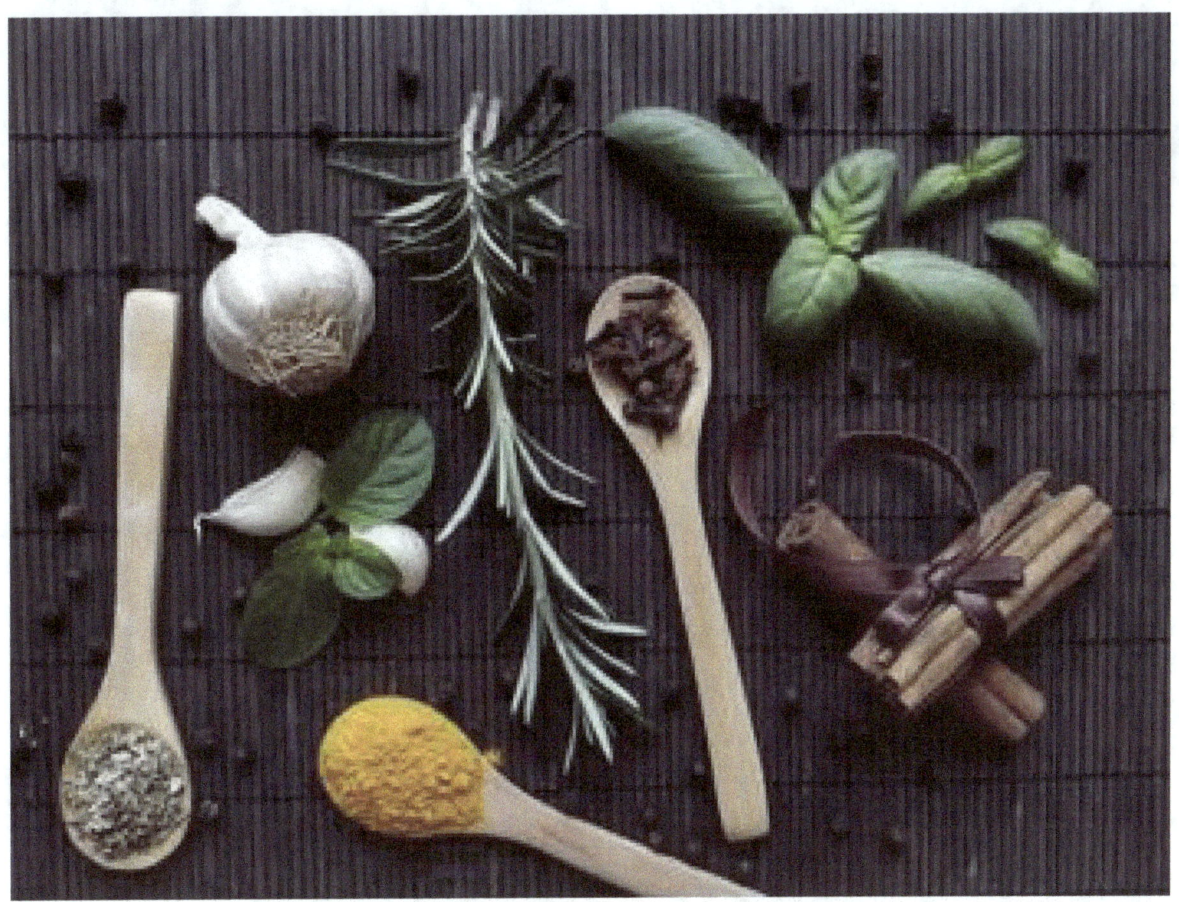

shutterstock.com · 1732478072

Spices such as oregano, cinnamon, and cloves contain antioxidants in the body. Lipoic acid, which is also in cinnamon, helps stimulate antioxidant production in the body and eliminate heavy metals that are responsible for oxidative stress.

"While lipoic is already present in the body, you can boost your intake through certain foods (like these aromatic spices."

Turmeric is used to help fight off inflammation but can be used to help protect against depression, arthritis and certain cancers.

-Watermelon

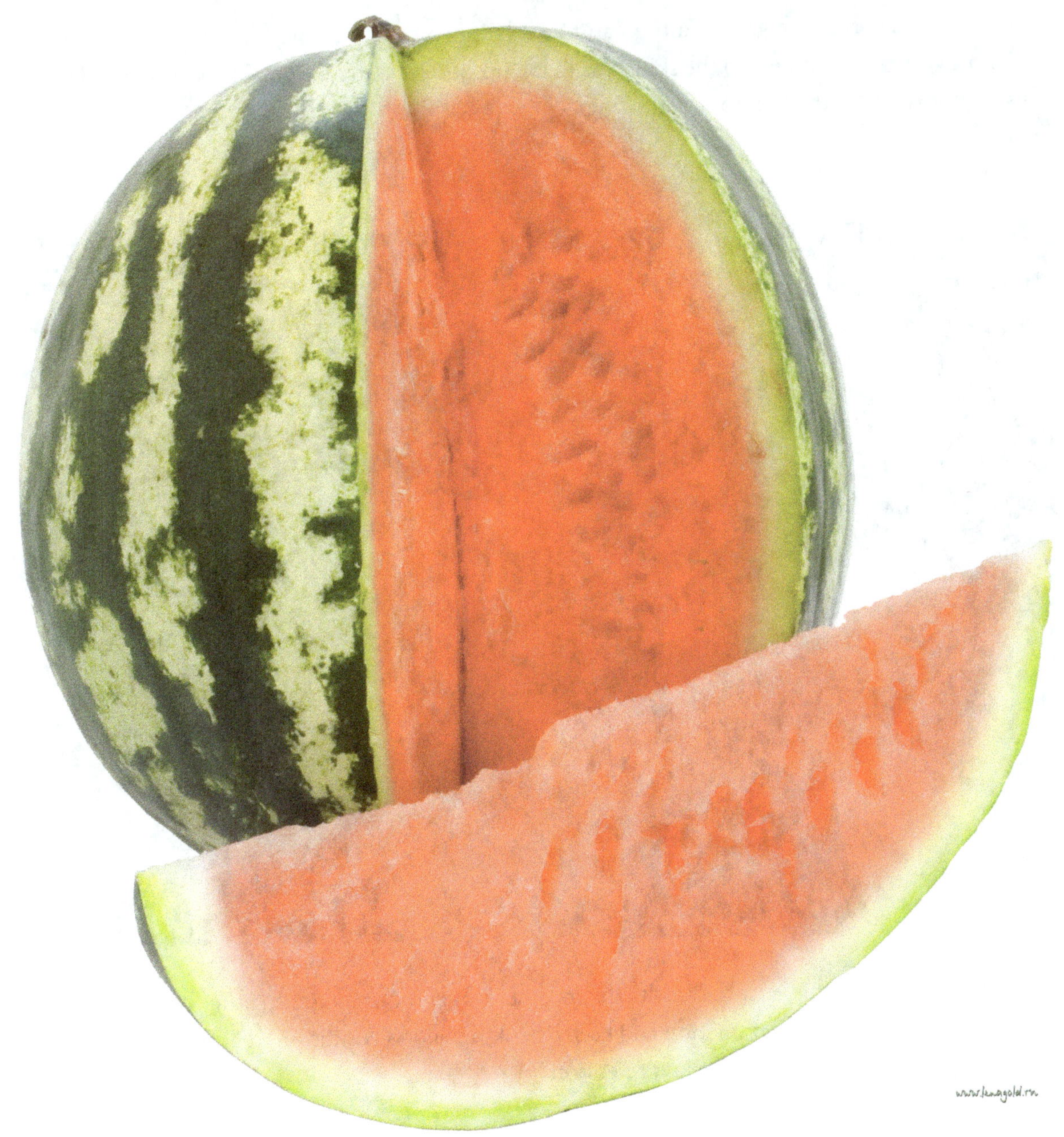

Watermelon contains high vitamins C and E. It helps to boost skin health along with lycopene which provides youthfulness to the skin. It is made up of 92% water and makes you stay hydrated. This is important for the skin to stay glowing.

-Walnut

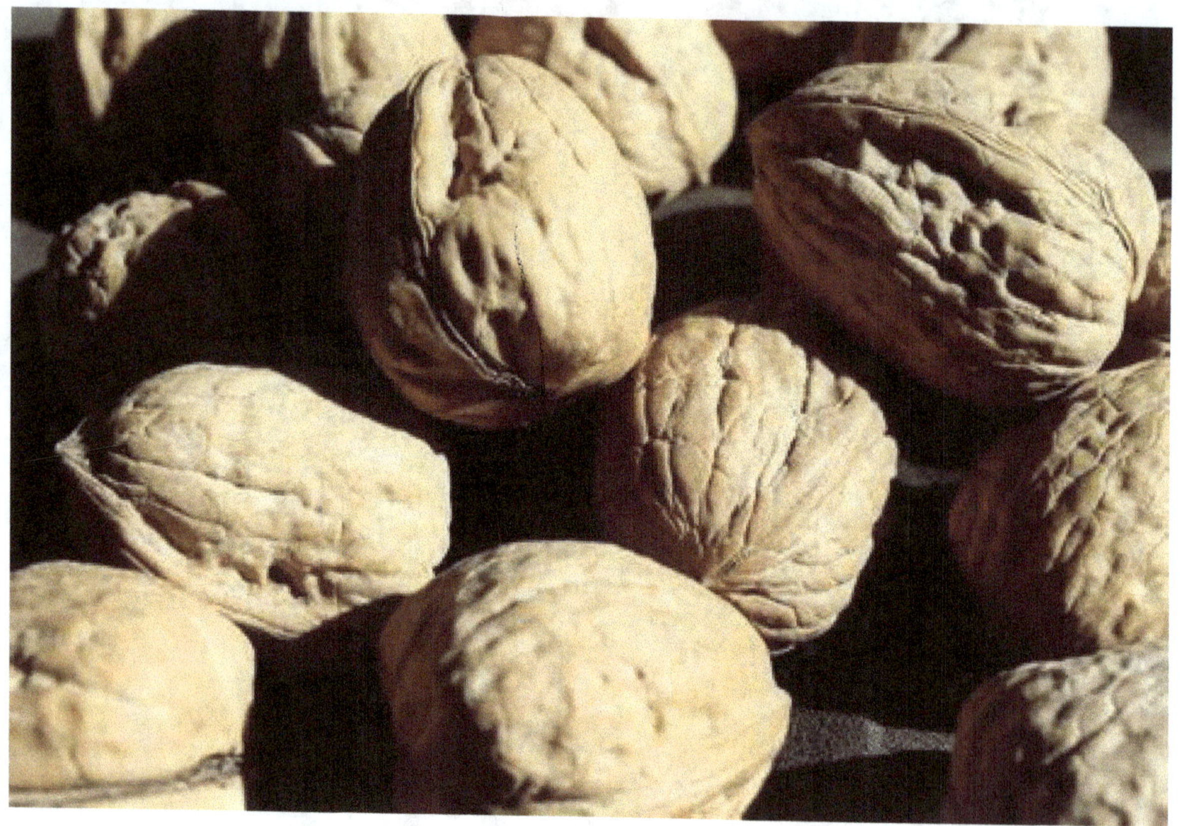

Walnuts contain more antioxidants than any other nut and carry a great source of omega-3 fats. It provides resistance to inflammation and keeps the skin in good condition. It also provides protection, temperature regulation and water retention.

-Grapes

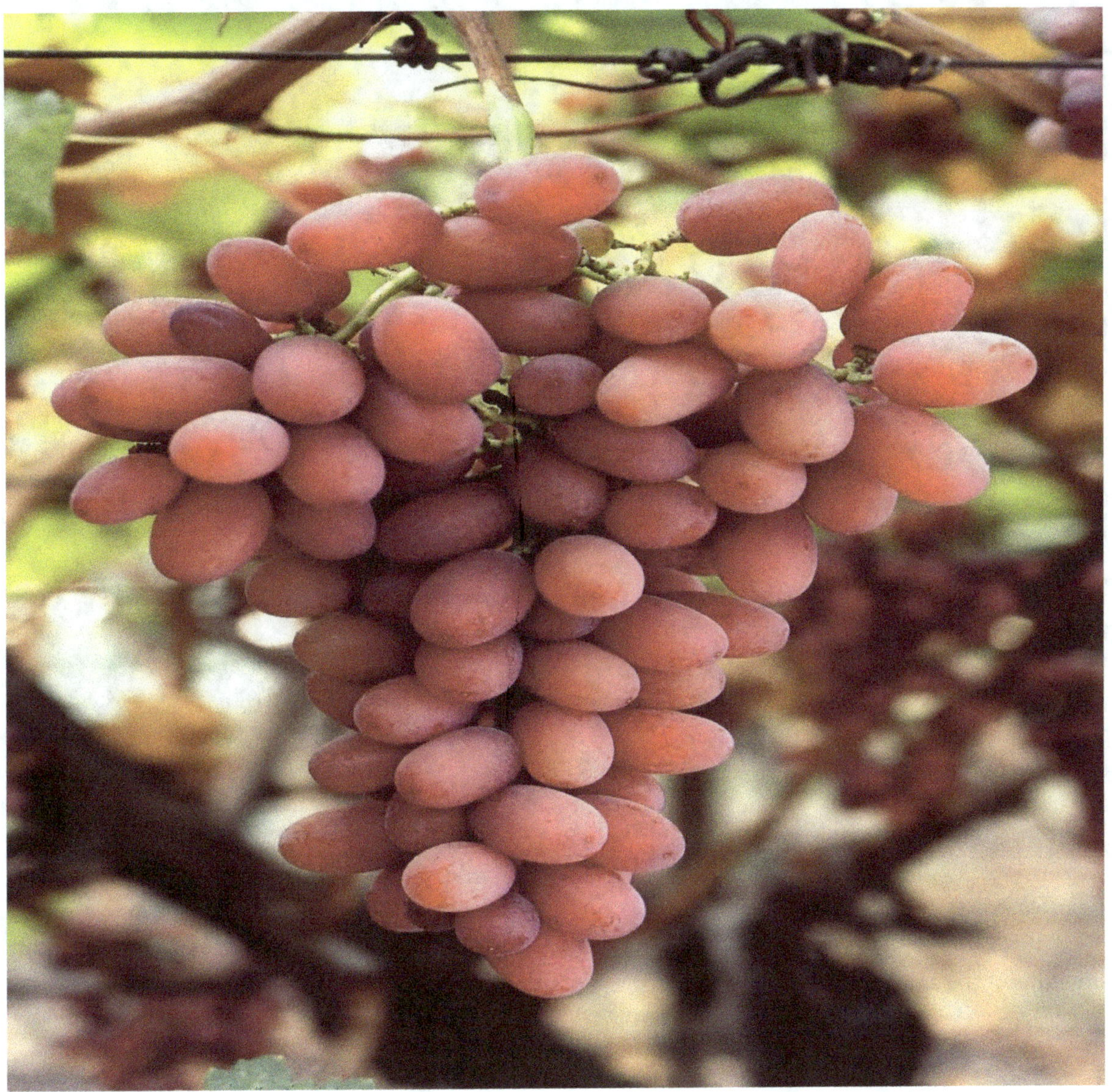

Grapes have antioxidants which are found in red wine. It is known to boost heart health. This antioxidant also protects collagen from free radicals and blood vessels. Collagen helps to protect the skin's elasticity, so the skin can stay glowing and vibrant for years to come.

Pomegranates

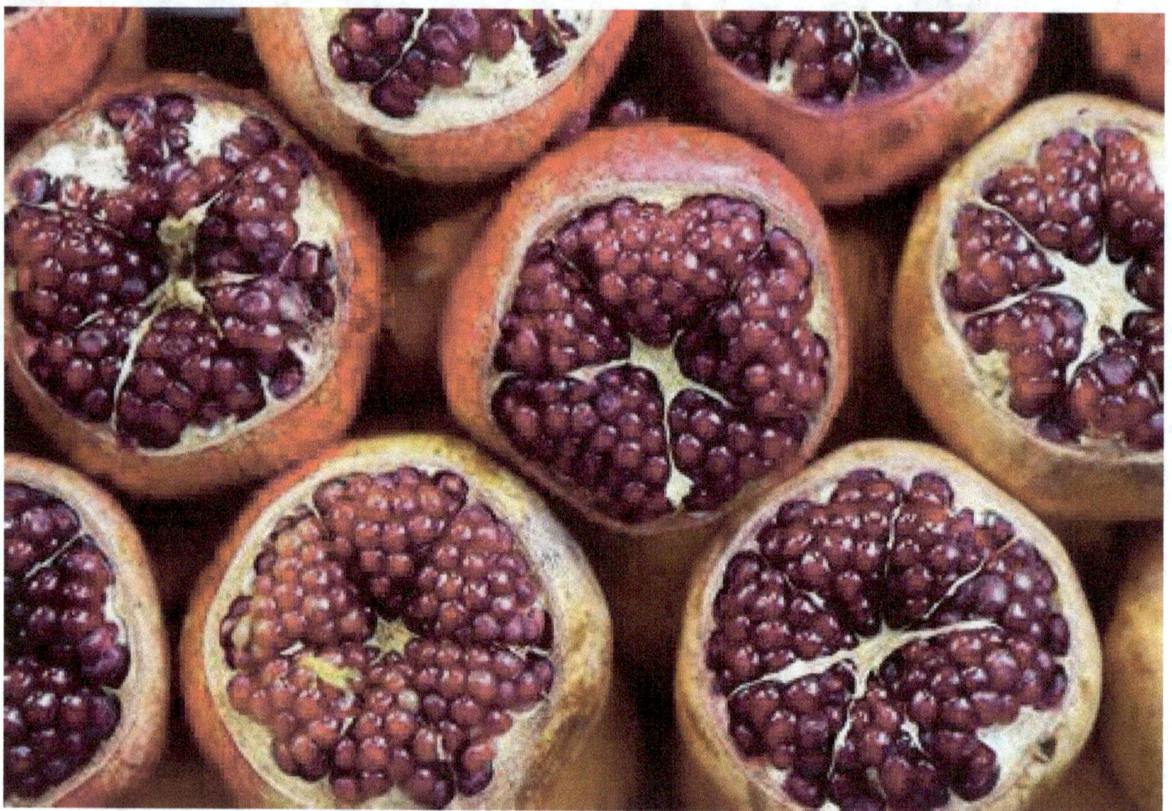

Pomegranates are loaded with allergic acid, and it can help prevent wrinkles. Pomegranates can slow down the aging process that can occur as a result of inflammation.

-Salmon

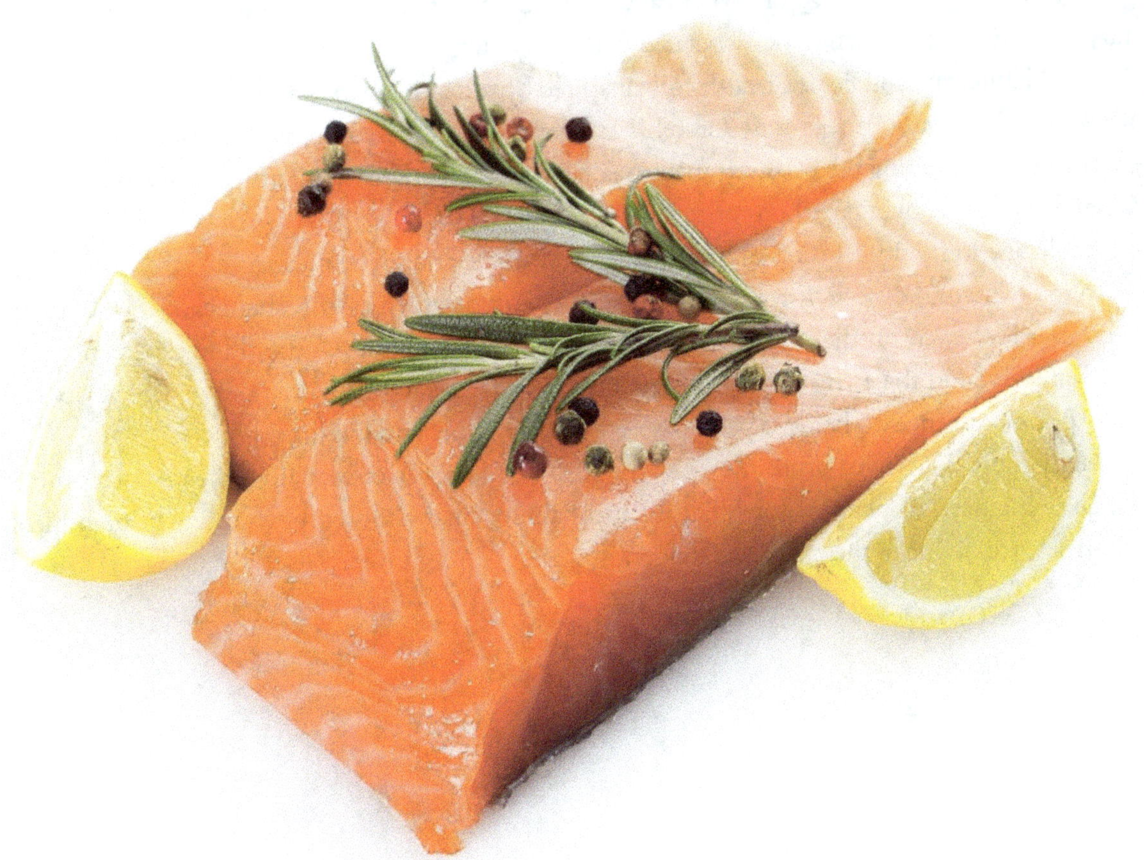

Salmon contains omega 3 and fatty fish like tuna and sardines, plus some shellfish like oysters. With all this combined, it would help you stay younger. This contains UV exposure that can act like a sunblock which helps to prevent sunburn.

In addition, the other factors would depend on how you eat, environment, activity level and social connection. Eating habits are the most important of all and would, in turn, lessen the doctors' visits and using medications. Medications have a lot of side effects that can affect other parts of your body, like your kidneys, liver, and heart. These can be problematic for a number of years to come.

Longer living is also based on a diet called 'The Mediterranean Diet', which is considered a dietary pattern that is known to be associated with longer living.

The Mediterranean Diet is a healthy diet inspired by the eating habits and traditional food typical of Southern Spain, Southern Italy Crete. It is a generic term based on traditional eating habits in the countries bordering the Mediterranean Sea. The diet is focused on plants and includes the traditional flavor and cooking methods of the region.

Achieving longevity requires major changes in your life and social norms.

In today's world expectations, the aging society concentrates more on changes in the population structure. However, on the longevity side, focus more on how they age and life expectancy gains. The longevity and the aging society, possess many challenges for a very long time. Longevity is the more popular of the two because people want to eat healthier and live longer.

Many individuals lived up to the 70's and 80's. Longevity stresses mainly the original problem, which is the need to plan for the 'plausible probability' that children born today in high-income countries, will live into their 90's and longer.

CHAPTER 2

Nutrition and diet

A healthy diet provides cells with vital energy sources and keeps them stable and working as they should; eating healthy foods boosts your immune cells. It fights against infections that are trying to affect the body and other health threats and also protects other cells from body damage. It also helps replace damaged cells.

Taking high sugars, unhealthy fats, and processed foods could cause damage and poor functions. Eating unhealthy foods like those mentioned above can cause increased infections, like cancers, inflammations, and chronic diseases such as diabetes, cardiovascular problems, and obesity.

Eating many fresh fruits and vegetables such as nuts, whole grains, legumes, and fish and minimizing red and processed meat were 23% less likely to die from and causes women who do not follow this dietary pattern. Balance diet, essential nutrients, superfoods, and meal planning.

Every day your 3 meals should include carbohydrates, fats, and proteins. The fiber would come from whole grains, fruits, and vegetables.

What to eat for a healthy balanced diet

A healthy diet generally includes a combination of the following:

Vegetables: Always a smart choice, aim to fill about half your plate with veggies. Add plenty of cruciferous veggies like broccoli and leafy greens, as well as colorful options like peppers.

◈ **Fruits:** Go for fresh fruit whenever possible and try various colors. Berries, grapes, apples, and grapefruits make great choices.

Whole grains: Eating grains in their whole form provides additional fiber and nutrients. This includes brown rice, oats, and 100% whole grain breads.

◇ **Lean protein:** High in protein and relatively low in fat, lean proteins include grilled chicken, ground turkey, and white fish.

◇ **Healthy fats:** Fatty fish, such as salmon and tuna, and nuts, such as walnuts, provide essential omega-3 fatty acids. Avocados are a great source of beneficial unsaturated fats.

7-Day Sample Menu

The one-week meal plan was designed for someone who needs about 2,000 to 2,2000 calories daily and has no dietary restrictions. Your daily calorie goal may vary. Learn what it is below, then tweak the plan to fit your specific needs. Consider working with a registered dietitian or speaking with a healthcare provider to assess and plan for your dietary needs more accurately.

Day 1
Breakfast

- One grapefruit
- Two eggs (or fried in a non-stick pan)
- One slice of 100% whole wheat toast

Macronutrients: approximately 327 calories, 18 grams of protein, 41 grams of carbohydrates, and 11 grams of fat
Snack

- One banana
- 1 cup plain yogurt with 1 tablespoon honey

Macronutrients: 324 calories, 14 grams protein, 62 grams carbohydrates, 4 grams fat
Lunch

- 6 ounces grille chicken breast

- Large garden salad (3 cups mixed greens with 1 cup cherry tomatoes, 1/4 avocado, topped with 2 tablespoons balsamic vinaigrette)

Macronutrients: 396 calories, 41 grams protein, 18 grams carbohydrates, 18 grams fat
Snack

- 1 cup (about 10) baby carrots
- 3 tablespoons hummus
- 1/2 piece of pita bread

Macronutrients: 192 calories, 7 grams protein, 31 grams carbohydrates, 5 grams fat
Dinner

- 1 cup steamed broccoli
- 1 cup of brown rice
- Halibut (4-ounce portion)

Macronutrients: 399 calories, 34 grams protein, 57 grams carbohydrates, 4 grams fat
Snack

- Two pitted Medjool dates
- 1 ounce 70% dark chocolate

Macronutrients: 302 calories, 3 grams protein, 49 grams carbohydrates, 12 grams fat
Daily Totals: *1,940 calories, 117 grams protein, 258 grams carbohydrates, 55 grams fat*
Note that beverages are not included in this meal plan. Individual fluid needs vary based on age, sex, activity level, and medical history. For optimal hydration, experts generally recommend drinking approximately 9 cups of water daily for women and 13 cups daily for men.[2] When adding beverages to your meal plan, consider their calorie count. Aim to reduce or eliminate consumption of sugar-sweetened beverages, and opt for water when possible.

Day 2
Breakfast

- One whole-wheat English muffin with 2 tablespoons of peanut butter
- One orange

Macronutrients: 391 calories with 14 grams of protein, 52 grams of carbohydrates, and 17 grams of fat

Snack

- One 7-ounce container of 2% plain Greek yogurt with 1/2 cup of blueberries

Macronutrients: 188 calories, 20 grams protein, 19grams carbohydrates, 4 grams fat

Lunch

- Turkey sandwich (6 ounces of turkey breast meat, large tomato slice, green lettuce, 1/4 avocado, and 2 teaspoons honey mustard on two slices of whole wheat bread)

Macronutrients: 540 calories, 59 grams protein, 34 grams carbohydrates, 18 grams fat

Snack

- 1 cup (about 30) grapes

Macronutrients: 100 calories, 1 grams protein, 27 grams carbohydrates, 0 grams fat

Dinner

- 5-ounce sirloin steak
- One roasted sweet potato
- 1 cup cooked spinach (made with 2 teaspoons olive oil)
- 1 cup green beans

Macronutrients: 612 calories, 48 grams protein, 40 grams carbohydrates, 30 grams fat
Snack

- 1 cup plain popcorn
- 1 ounce 70% dark chocolate

Macronutrients: Approximately 214 calories, 2.9 grams protein, 17 grams carbohydrates, 3 grams fat

Daily Totals: *2,045 calories, 145 grams protein, 188 grams carbohydrates, 85 grams fat*
Day 3
Breakfast

- Overnight Oats (one mashed banana, 2 tablespoons chia seeds, 1/2 cup oats, 1 cup almond milk, 1 teaspoon cinnamon)

Macronutrients: approximately 431 calories with 12 grams protein, 73 grams carbohydrates, 13 grams fat
Snack

- One fresh pear
- 1 ounce (22) almonds

Macronutrients: 271 calories, 7 grams protein, 33 grams carbohydrates, 15 grams fat
Lunch

- One fried egg
- One slice whole-wheat bread
- 1/2 avocado, mashed
- 1 medium apple

Macronutrients: 408 calories, 13 grams protein, 48 grams carbohydrates, 21 grams fat
Snack

- 3 tablespoons hummus
- 1 cup baby carrots
- 1 cup cherry tomatoes

Macronutrients: 140 calories, 6 grams protein, 21 grams carbohydrates, 5 grams fat
Dinner

- One whole wheat English muffin
- One slice tomato, two leaves lettuce, one slice onion
- 5-ounce turkey burger
- 2 tablespoons ketchup

Macronutrients: 531 calories, 43 grams protein, 38 grams carbohydrates, 24 grams fat
Snack

- 1 cup of ice cream
- 1 cup fresh raspberries

Macronutrients: 337 calories, 6 grams protein, 46 grams carbohydrates, 15 grams fat
Daily Totals: *2,118 calories, 86 grams protein, 259 grams carbohydrates, 93 grams fat*
Day 4
Breakfast

- Two slices 100% whole wheat toast with 2 tablespoons peanut butter
- One banana

Macronutrients: approximately 454 calories with 16 grams of protein, 62 grams of carbohydrates, and 18 grams of fat

Snack

- 1 cup grapes
- 1 ounce (14) walnuts

Macronutrients: 290 calories, 5 grams protein, 31 grams carbohydrates, 19 grams fat

Lunch

- Tuna wrap with one wheat flour tortilla, 1/2 can water-packed tuna (drained), 1 tablespoon mayonnaise, lettuce, and sliced tomato
- 1/2 sliced avocado

Macronutrients: 496 calories, 27 grams protein, 28 grams carbohydrates, 132grams fat

Snack

- 1 cup cottage cheese (1% fat)
- 1/2 cup blueberries

Macronutrients: 205 calories, 29 grams protein, 17 grams carbohydrates, 3 grams fat

Dinner

- 1 1/2 cups whole wheat pasta
- 1 cup tomato sauce
- Small garden salad (1 cup mixed greens with one half cup cherry tomatoes topped with one tablespoon balsamic vinaigrette)

Macronutrients: 472 calories, 18 grams protein, 91 grams carbohydrates, 8 grams fat

Snack

- One apple

Macronutrients: 95 calories, 0.5 grams protein, 25 grams carbohydrates, 0.3 grams fat
Daily Totals: *2,012 calories, 96 grams protein, 255 grams carbohydrates, 80 grams fat*
Day 5
Breakfast

- One whole wheat bagel
- 3 tablespoons cream cheese

Macronutrients: approximately 441 calories with 15 grams of protein, 59 grams of carbohydrates, and 16 grams of fat
Snack

- 1 cup baby carrots
- 1 cup cauliflower pieces
- 2 tablespoons ranch dressing

Macronutrients: 191 calories, 3 grams protein, 15 grams carbohydrates, 14 grams fat
Lunch

- Veggie burger
- Whole grain bun
- One slice of cheddar cheese
- One sliced apple

Macronutrients: 573 calories, 25 grams protein, 62 grams carbohydrates, 26 grams fat
Snack

- One banana
- 2 tablespoons peanut butter

Macronutrients: 293 calories, 8 grams protein, 35 grams carbohydrates, 16 grams fat
Dinner

- 4 ounces trout filet
- 1 cup steamed green beans
- 1 cup brown rice
- One small garden salad with 1 tablespoon of salad dressing

Macronutrients: 526 calories, 38 grams protein, 60 grams carbohydrates, 15 grams fat
Snack

- One fresh peach

Macronutrients: 68 calories, 2 grams protein, 17 grams carbohydrates, 0.4 grams fat)
Daily Totals: *2,092 calories, 90 grams protein, 249 grams carbohydrates, 88 grams fat*
Day 6
Breakfast

- One (7-ounce) container of 2% Greek yogurt
- One banana
- One hard-boiled egg

Macronutrients: approximately 323calories with 27 grams protein, 35 grams carbohydrates, and 9 grams fat
Snack

- 10 whole wheat pretzel twists

- 3 tablespoons hummus

Macronutrients: 305 calories, 10 grams protein, 55 grams carbohydrates, 6 grams fat
Lunch

- One whole wheat tortilla
- 4 ounces turkey
- One slice of cheddar cheese
- 1 cup mixed greens
- 1 tablespoon honey mustard

Macronutrients: 531 calories, 43 grams protein, 25 grams carbohydrates, 28 grams fat
Snack

- 1/2 ounce (11) almonds
- One fresh peach

Macronutrients: 153 calories, 5 grams protein, 20 grams carbohydrates, 8 grams fat
Dinner

- 5 ounces pork loin
- Small garden salad with 1 tablespoon vinaigrette
- 1 medium baked sweet potato
- 5 asparagus spears

Macronutrients: 440 calories, 42 grams protein, 31 grams carbohydrates, 16 grams fat
Snack

- One medium chocolate chip cookie
- 1 cup sliced strawberries

Macronutrients: 201 calories, 3 grams protein, 32 grams carbohydrates, 8 grams fat
Daily Totals: *1,952 calories, 130 grams protein, 198 grams carbohydrates, 75 grams fat*

Day 7

Breakfast

- 1 cup cooked oatmeal
- 1/2 cup blueberries
- 1/2 cup non-fat milk
- 2 tablespoons almond butter

Macronutrients: 439 calories, 17 grams protein, 50 grams carbohydrates, 21 grams fat

Snack

- One (7-ounce) container of 2% Greek yogurt
- One sliced apple

Macronutrients: 241 calories, 20 grams protein, 33 grams carbohydrates, 4 grams fat

Lunch

- 6-ounce baked chicken breast
- Large garden salad with tomatoes and onions and 2 tablespoons of balsamic vinaigrette
- One baked sweet potato

Macronutrients: 708 calories, 45 grams protein, 42 grams carbohydrates, 40 grams fat

Snack

- 1 cup raw broccoli florets
- 1 cup baby carrots
- 3 tablespoons hummus

Macronutrients: 168 calories, 8 grams protein, 26 grams carbohydrates, 6 grams fat
Dinner

- A 4-ounce serving of baked or grilled salmon
- 1 cup brown rice
- Five asparagus spears

Macronutrients: 468 calories, 31 grams protein, 49 grams carbohydrates, 16 grams fat
Snack

- One peach

(Macronutrients: 68 calories, 2 grams protein, 17 grams carbohydrates, 0 grams fat)
Daily Totals: *2,093 calories, 124 grams protein, 218 grams carbohydrates, 86 grams fat*

Exercise and Longevity

A multitude of studies show that physical activity contributes to greater longevity due to the many positive effects it has on the body. These effects include stronger heart and lung function, improved health of blood vessels, stronger muscles, better balance, and a healthier weight. (' Havard University)

Being more active may lower your risk of heart attack, stroke, falling, and diabetes, among other benefits. Together, these benefits contribute to a longer lifespan. Physical activity can also improve your mood and help you sleep better.

This is how much you need to stay physically fit and to add some age to your life

- 150 minutes a week of moderate activity
- 75 minutes a week of vigorous movement or
- An equivalent combination of both intensities

Moderate physical activity includes walking, weight lifting, and lower-intensity exercises. Vigorous exercise includes running, bicycling, and swimming. Even household tasks like cleaning and gardening count as exercise. So does lifting small hand weights or doing leg lifts while watching TV. The guidelines also recommend muscle-strengthening activities on two or more days per week.

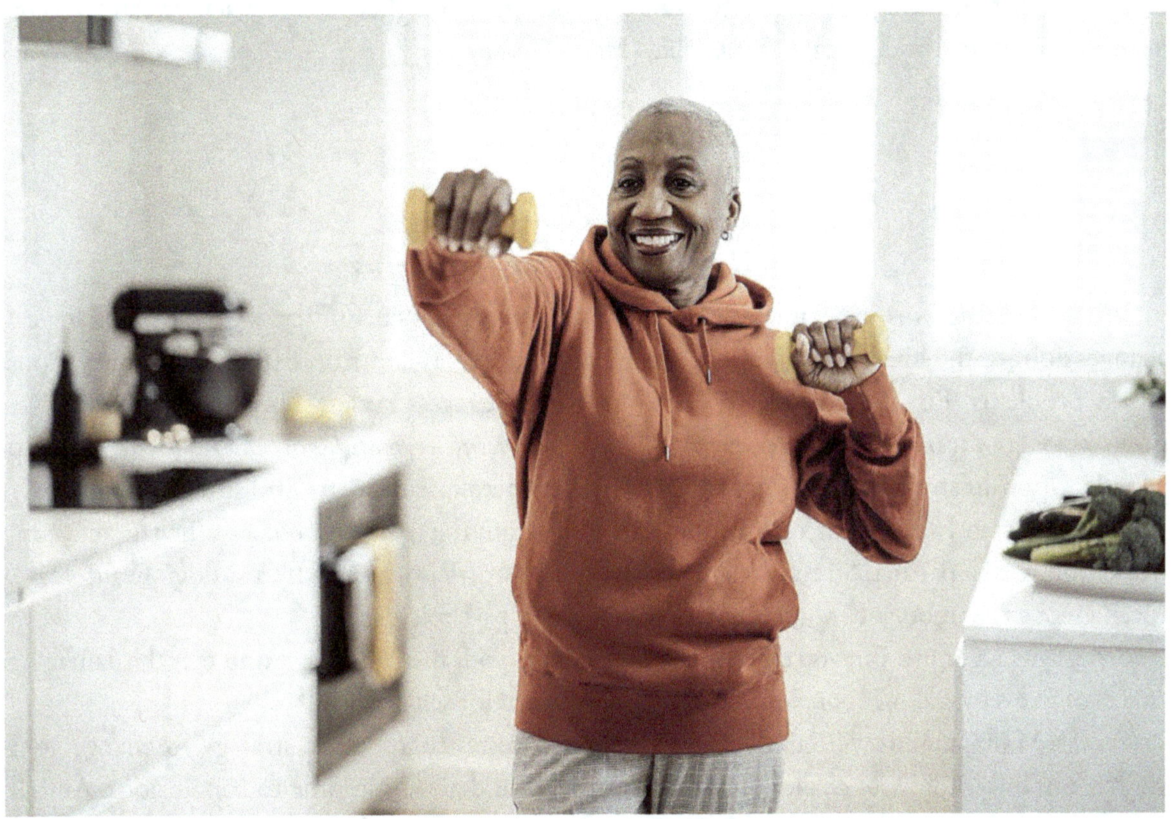

Heart-pumping exercise goes a long way toward achieving robust health, but adding strength training to your regimen may be key to living even longer. That's the finding of a large study published online Oct. 17, 2022, by *JAMA Network Open*. Researchers evaluated physical activity reported by more than 115,000 people ages 65 and older as part of the ongoing National Health Interview Survey. They compared exercise data with deaths over an average of nearly eight years. Regardless of how much aerobic exercise they did, participants who did strength training two to six times weekly were less likely to die from any cause during the study period compared with those who did less strength training. People who did at least two strength training sessions and 2.5 hours of moderate-to-vigorous aerobic activity each week were 30% less likely to die during that time. The observational study did not prove conclusively that doing strength training or aerobic exercise caused people to live longer. Strength training includes lifting weights, using resistance bands, doing push-ups or sit-ups, or digging in the garden. (Heidi Godman)

Mental and Emotional Well-being

While some stress is inevitable, when your body repeatedly encounters a set of physiological changes dubbed the stress response, trouble can brew. Stress may contribute to or exacerbate various health problems. But it's possible to dismantle negative stress cycles. This Special Health Report, *Stress Management: Enhance your well-being by reducing stress and building resilience,* can help you identify your stress warning signs and learn how to better manage stressful situations.

Stress constantly creeps into our lives. It can come from the frustration of a traffic jam or a confrontation with a partner. Stress can spurred by money worries or spiked by a sudden health scare. It can exact a toll upon you- physically, emotionally, and psychologically.

Stress is a fact of life. But you determine how it affects your life. You can counteract the damaging effects of stress by calling upon your body's rich potential for self-healing.

Stress Management will help you explore cognitive restructuring, a strategy to change your views. You'll learn how to challenge negative thoughts and avoid jumping to conclusions. And, if you've heard about the power of visualization and meditation but don't know where to start, the report will show you.

Everyone worries or gets scared sometimes. But if you feel extremely worried or afraid much of the time, or if you repeatedly feel panicky, you may have an anxiety disorder. Anxiety disorders are among the most common mental illnesses, affecting roughly 40 million American adults each year. This Special Health Report, *Anxiety, and Stress Disorders,* discusses the latest and most effective treatment approaches, including cognitive behavioral therapies, psychotherapy, and medications. A special section delves into alternative treatments for anxiety, such as relaxation techniques, mindfulness meditation, and biofeedback.

Cognitive behavioral therapy (CBT), the leading form of therapy for anxiety, aims to correct ingrained patterns of negative thoughts and behaviors. As the name suggests, it has two parts. Cognitive therapy helps people change patterns of thinking that prevent them from overcoming their fears. Behavioral therapy works to change their reactions in situations that trigger anxiety.

People with social phobia, for example, may assume that others will inevitably regard what they say as stupid. This is negative thinking. As a result, these people may avoid being with or talking to others. This is an example of negative behavior. The goal of CBT is to break this chain of thoughts and reactions.

Because negative thoughts and behaviors tend to come to the fore when people are under stress, the first step in CBT is to help you recognize when you're stressed. It's important to have an inner "thermostat" that can tell you how stressed you are and how to dial it down.

Behavioral therapists say there are three components to a stress reaction. These are commonly called the ABCs: affect, behavior, and cognition. Affect is how you feel; it refers to your emotional response to a situation. Behavior is what you do; for example, it can include tensing your jaw, tapping your foot, pacing, or overeating. Cognition refers to your thoughts when stressed; for example, thinking, "I'm going to miss my work deadline and get fired."

Research has shown that CBT is effective for panic disorder, generalized anxiety disorder, post-traumatic stress disorder, specific phobia, and social phobia. CBT can be done individually or in a group. If the anxiety is the result of a traumatic event that affected more than one person, group therapy may be most effective.

CBT usually takes place weekly for several weeks or months; once your condition stabilizes, you may see the doctor once or twice a month or only if symptoms worsen.

The therapist typically begins by asking you to record your thoughts and level of anxiety in certain situations. Then, you and the therapist discuss these thoughts, evaluate their reality, and work together to substitute more productive thoughts. The therapist might also challenge you to consider what would happen if the fears came true and whether that outcome would be so bad.

The behavioral component of CBT incorporates two main strategies. The first, called exposure or desensitization, involves people facing their fears directly. This can be done in several ways. One is through role-playing. Another is by having a person imagine frightening situations and describe them. Yet another strategy is to give people "homework" in which they put themselves in real-life situations that spark anxiety. The reasoning is that avoiding anxiety-causing thoughts and situations reinforces fears or false beliefs. In real-life situations, people can practice recognizing negative thoughts and substituting more realistic ones. With repeated exposure, people eventually become desensitized to fear-provoking situations.

The other main strategy is teaching people practical skills to help them feel more in control in difficult situations. For those who become extremely anxious when they have much to do, this may mean offering tips on setting goals and managing time. Those uneasy in social situations can be coached in conversational techniques and other social skills.

CHAPTER 3

Social Relationships

Two decades of research indicate causal associations between social relationships and mortality, but important questions remain regarding how social relationships affect health when effects emerge, and how long they last. Drawing on data from four nationally representative longitudinal samples of the US population, we implemented an innovative life course design to assess the prospective association of both structural and functional dimensions of social relationships (social integration, social support, and social strain) with objectively measured biomarkers of physical health (C-reactive protein, systolic and diastolic blood pressure, waist circumference, and body mass index) within each life stage, including adolescence and young, middle, and late adulthood, and compare such associations across life stages. We found that a higher degree of social integration was associated with a lower risk of physiological dysregulation in a dose-response manner in both early and later life. Conversely, lack of social connections was associated with vastly elevated risk in specific life stages. For example, social isolation increased the risk of inflammation by the same magnitude as physical inactivity in adolescence, and the effect of social isolation on hypertension exceeded that of clinical risk factors such as diabetes in old age. Analyses of multiple dimensions of social relationships within multiple samples across the life course produced consistent and robust associations with health. Physiological impacts of structural and functional dimensions of social relationships emerge uniquely in adolescence and midlife and persist into old age.

A defining characteristic of human society is that individual lives are intertwined through social relationships. Full social participation is such a fundamental human need that research since the 1900s has found the lack of social connections increases the odds of death by at least 50%. When multidimensional assessments of social relationships were considered, the odds of mortality increased by 91% among the socially isolated. The magnitude of this effect is comparable to that of smoking and exceeds those of many other known risk factors of mortality, such as obesity or physical inactivity. Although much evidence has accrued on the strong causal associations between social relationships and mortality as well as other health outcomes, important questions remain as to how social relationships affect health, when these effects emerge, and how long they last

Studies of social, psychological, and behavioral mechanisms underlying the social relationship gradient in health have shed light on the first question. It is less clear, however, what biological mechanisms may be at play. Recent research on the biology of aging emphasizes the essential role of physiological stress response and regulation across multiple bodily systems in shaping longevity. Although social relationship gradients in health and longevity path and physiological determinants of mortality have been widely documented, these separate bodies of research have yet to be fully integrated. We have yet to determine whether social relationship differentials in longevity arise from a biological process in which social experiences "get under the skin" to alter physiological regulatory systems.

Examining how social and biological processes unfold and interact as individuals age is a critical step in advancing scientific explanations of the emergence and progression of diseases. A life course perspective, represented by the horizontal arrow D as a developmental trajectory, has not been fully brought to bear on this question. This perspective may offer considerable leverage by linking physical risks to social exposures across multiple developmental stages from early to late life. The vast majority of biosocial research to date on this association has focused on older adults for whom morbidity and mortality rates are high. However, early life social experiences may be biologically embedded at that time, as shown by an increasing body of research linking childhood disadvantage and maltreatment to an increased likelihood of exaggerated biological stress response and, in turn, higher risks of inflammation and cardiovascular disease throughout adulthood.

Relationship deficits—such as social isolation, lack of support, or high strain—are alternative forms of social adversity that can create chronic stress by continuous exposure to chains of risk that accumulate over the life course. Individuals who experience early adversity are subject to multiple and longer durations of stress exposure and are more prone to inflammatory and stress-related diseases as they age. At the same time, the emergence of chronic diseases usually takes many decades due to the long latency after the initial risk exposures. Therefore, extensive longitudinal data and analyses are imperative to understanding how the connection of social relationships and longevity unfolds over the human life span. Little empirical research depicts this lifelong process partly because data that extend sufficiently over long periods of the life course, are exceedingly rare.

We make three unique contributions that shed new light on the social aspects of longevity. First, using data from an array of nationally representative longitudinal samples of the US population, we implement an innovative life course design that begins at the earliest developmental stage (adolescence) in which physiological consequences of key social relationship patterns begin to manifest and trace subsequent life stages (young, middle, late adulthood) to depict the life-long process of stress response cascades that such relationship patterns initiate. The data come from The National Longitudinal Study of Adolescent to Adult Health (Add Health) to capture adolescence and young adulthood, the National Survey of Midlife Development in the United States (MIDUS) for middle adulthood, and both the Health and Retirement Study (HRS) and the National Social Life, Health, and Aging Project (NSHAP) for late adulthood. Using multiple large, population-based samples in an integrative design allows us to assess linkages between social relationships and health for each life stage. It also offers an unprecedented fuller view of age variations in such linkages than any previous study of a particular sample or single life stage alone. Second, this study uses comprehensive and refined measurements of social relationships that encompass two primary dimensions that may differentially influence physical health at different stages of the life course. It assesses measures of social integration to capture the structural–quantitative dimension and measures of social support and strain to capture the functional–qualitative dimension, using age-appropriate conceptualizations of these domains for each life stage. Third, the study examines multiple objectively measured biomarkers or endophenotypes, including inflammation (C-reactive protein, CRP), cardiovascular function (hypertension), and energy metabolism (overall obesity and abdominal obesity) to capture key physiological mechanisms underlying common diseases of aging and longevity.

CHAPTER 4

Sleep and Restoration

Ticking away in the shadows of our pillows, a silent clock governs the delicate balance between vibrant longevity and premature decline. This invisible timekeeper, known as our sleep cycle, plays a crucial role in determining not only the quality of our daily lives but also the length of our overall lifespan. As we delve into the intricate relationship between sleep and longevity, we uncover a fascinating web of biological processes, scientific discoveries, and lifestyle factors that collectively shape our journey through life.

The connection between sleep and longevity has garnered increasing attention in recent years as researchers uncover more evidence linking adequate rest to a longer, healthier life. Current statistics paint a concerning picture of global sleep habits, with many individuals falling short of recommended sleep durations. According to recent studies, approximately one-third of adults in developed countries regularly experience insufficient sleep, a trend that correlates with reduced life expectancy. This growing body of research has propelled sleep science to the forefront of health and longevity studies, prompting scientists to explore the intricate mechanisms through which sleep influences our overall well-being and lifespan.

The Science Behind Sleep and Life Expectancy

At the heart of the sleep-longevity connection lies a complex interplay of cellular processes during our nightly slumber. While we rest, our bodies engage in a remarkable feat of repair and regeneration, working tirelessly to maintain and restore our physical and mental faculties. This restorative process is fundamental to our long-term health and plays a significant role in determining our lifespan.

One of the primary ways sleep affects our longevity is through its impact on cellular repair. During deep sleep stages, our bodies produce higher levels of growth hormone, which is essential for tissue repair and cell regeneration. This hormone helps to repair damage caused by daily wear and tear, oxidative stress, and environmental factors. Without adequate sleep, our cells may accumulate damage over time, potentially leading to accelerated aging and increased susceptibility to age-related diseases.

Moreover, sleep is crucial in hormone regulation and metabolism, intricately linked to our overall health and longevity. During sleep, our bodies regulate the production of various hormones, including cortisol (the stress hormone), leptin, and ghrelin (hunger hormones). Disruptions in sleep patterns can lead to imbalances in these hormones, potentially contributing to weight gain, metabolic disorders, and increased stress levels – all of which can negatively impact our lifespan.

CHAPTER 5

Lifelong Learning and Cognitive Health

Embarking on a journey of **lifelong learning** may seem like an overwhelming task. However, the potential benefits for **brain health and cognitive function** are profound. Engaging in continuous learning activities can positively impact various aspects of brain function, ultimately improving overall mental abilities.

Research has shown that **lifelong learning** can contribute to a lower risk of developing age-related cognitive decline and dementia. Additionally, **challenging the brain** with new information and skills can help to build and strengthen neural connections, ultimately enhancing mental function. Actively seeking opportunities for lifelong learning can improve memory, attention, and problem-solving skills, leading to a better quality of life in old age.

- **Continuous learning:** Engaging in lifelong learning activities such as reading, puzzles, and new skills can help keep the brain active and healthy.
- **Enhanced cognitive function:** Lifelong learning can enhance cognitive function and reduce dementia risk.
- **Improved overall brain health:** Regular mental stimulation through lifelong learning can promote the growth of new brain cells, strengthen neural connections, and enhance cognitive reserve.

CHAPTER 6

Preventive Healthcare and Regular Check-ups

Some healthcare leaders have called for an end to annual health check visits, saying they're a waste of time for patients and overworked primary care physicians and don't reduce the risk of death.

A new Northwestern Medicine study published in *JAMA* has found that while there is no clear proof that regular check-ups help adults live longer or prevent cardiovascular events like heart attacks or strokes, they still have many health benefits – especially for at-risk populations – and should continue.

Routine check-up visits (they don't have to necessarily be done annually) can lead to better detection and treatment of chronic illnesses such as depression and hypertension, an increase in vaccinations and screenings for diseases like cancer, and improve how a patient feels after visiting with a doctor (patient-reported outcomes), the study found.

"While it is disappointing that I can't tell my patients a visit with me or my colleagues will help them live longer, it is good to know there are proven, measurable benefits," said senior study author Jeffrey Linder, '97 MD, MPH, chief of General Internal Medicine and Geriatrics in the Department of Medicine and a Northwestern Medicine physician.

The study is a review of 32 studies conducted between 1963 and 2021.

"I was surprised at how many benefits we found when we dug into the data, given the negative messaging around these exams," said first study author David Liss, PhD, research associate professor of Medicine in the Division of General Internal Medicine and Geriatrics. "Especially when it relates to patient-reported outcomes. If you walk away feeling healthy, it becomes a self-fulfilling prophecy.

"I think many of the critics meant to say 'Don't do these annual exams for low-risk patients,' but the message came out to not do these exams at all, which is problematic."

'Sick visits' don't allow for all the necessary screenings.

For at-risk populations, these exams are still vital, Liss said. They include patients who are ethnic or racial minorities, overdue for preventive services, and have uncontrolled risk factors, such as diet, exercise, and smoking; low self-rated health; don't have a single source of trusted care; or live in geographic areas with low access to primary care providers.

"A lot of people only see a doctor when there is a problem," Liss said. "But that often doesn't leave time to discuss vaccinations or cancer screenings. It's easy to see the value in routine check-ups because there are multiple recommended services that could be discussed in these visits."

Cost should not be a factor because every patient with Medicare coverage and many insured patients 65 years and older can get an annual wellness visit for $0 copay, Liss said.

The study examined a variety of factors, including mortality (risk of premature death) and cardiovascular outcomes (heart attacks or heart disease), which did not benefit from general health checks.

However, several remaining factors saw added benefits from routine check-ups, including chronic disease detection (e.g. increases in statin or depression prescriptions); risk factor control (improved blood pressure, cholesterol readings); clinical preventive services (more screenings and vaccinations); and patient-reported outcomes.

'The patient is the only person who knows how they feel'

Physicians are increasingly discussing "patient-reported outcomes" or "self-reported outcomes" as a measure of someone's health, almost equivalent to lab results or scan readings.

"It speaks to peoples' states of mind," Liss said. "There's a general sense of health when they walk away from these visits, maybe thinking, 'Hey, I'm not as unhealthy as I thought I was.' The patient is the only person who knows how they feel. The feelings people carry with them are important to their health and wellbeing over time."

Seeing a consistent and trusted source of primary care is important to foster relationships and makes it easier to reach out to doctors when there is a problem, Liss said, adding that just talking to someone about your concerns can make you feel better.

CHAPTER 7

The Role of Technology and Innovation in Aging

Older adults rapidly adopted technology for healthcare, known as digital health, during the COVID-19 pandemic. Older adults increasingly use telehealth, smartphone apps, and other digital health technologies to reduce barriers to care, maintain patient-provider communication, and promote disease self-management. Yet, many healthcare professionals have maintained outdated beliefs rooted in societal ageism that digital health and older adults are incompatible. As a result, older adults have been disproportionally excluded from health services and clinical trials that use digital health relative to their younger counterparts. In this commentary, we urge all healthcare disciplines to challenge ageist beliefs and practices contributing to the "digital health divide" among older patients. We provide examples of evidence-based strategies and current scientific initiatives that can promote digital health inclusion in research, clinical practice, and training. By achieving digital health inclusion, we can increase access, provide preventative and comprehensive care, and decrease healthcare costs for older patients.

Keywords: Digital health, Technology, Access to care, Interdisciplinary, Public health

In this commentary, we urge all healthcare disciplines to challenge ageist beliefs and practices contributing to the "digital health divide" among older patients. By achieving digital health inclusion, we can increase access, provide preventative and comprehensive care, and decrease healthcare costs for older patients.

RAPID GROWTH OF DIGITAL HEALTH

Consumer technology is ubiquitous in modern society and is increasingly embraced by older adults (age ≥ 65). The number of older adults who own a smartphone has risen dramatically from 18% in 2013 to 83% (age 50–64) and 61% (age 65+) in 2021. An even larger portion of older adults own a laptop or computer (90%) and use the internet. As people live longer, technologies become more affordable, and broadband access increases, we can expect that the prevalence of "plugged-in" older adults will continue to rise. Technology in healthcare, known as digital health, has proliferated in many forms, including mobile health, health information technology, wearable devices, telehealth, and personalized medicine. Digital health offers a promising solution to improve medical outcomes and enhance the efficiency of healthcare for all individuals, including older adults.

Upward trends of digital health adoption by older adults were further accelerated by the COVID-19 pandemic. The number of older adults (age ≥ 70) who completed telehealth visits with their provider increased to 21.1% from 4.6% pre-pandemic. Older adults have also engaged with digital coaching platforms that promote disease self-management and lifestyle changes at rates that exceed younger patients. Digital health has provided a safe alternative to in-person visits for vulnerable and home-bound patients, reduced travel burden, and facilitated provider communication. For these reasons, older adults increasingly view digital health as essential; however, many healthcare professionals remain reluctant.

AGEIST BELIEFS AND PRACTICES IN DIGITAL HEALTH

Ageism has deep roots in our society, and it negatively impacts older patients Common ageist beliefs (e.g., *"you can't teach an old dog new tricks"*) in healthcare can lead to harmful generalizations that all older adults are unwilling or unable to use technology. In a recent qualitative interview study, healthcare professionals equated older age with poor technological skills and endorsed a lack of competence of digital health competence As a result, clinicians may be unprepared to implement digital health into practice, recommend digital health treatments to older patients, and tailor technologies to their specific needs. In research, older adults are excluded from clinical trials due to advanced age, medical comorbidities, and concerns regarding technology use. Institutional barriers, such as the design of patient portals, deter older adults from accessing health information. As a result, older adults risk becoming underrepresented in digital health at all levels of healthcare.

Generalizations that older adults are technologically incompetent to disregard the complex biopsychosocial factors that contribute to digital health exclusion. These factors can include visual and hearing impairment, physical disability, speech-language difficulties, cognitive impairment, lack of familiarity with technology, and not owning devices. Older adults with lower income, remote or rural residences, and medical complexities face even greater obstacles in using and accessing digital health. In a survey of home-bound older adults during COVID-19, Black non-Hispanic and Hispanic/Latino individuals had the lowest rates of digital health. Disparities in access and prior negative experiences with technology, along with the lack of support from healthcare professionals, can make some older adults less likely to adopt digital health and ask for help. Over 10 million older Americans are not ready to use digital health due are a result of these biopsychosocial factors. A new approach is needed to prevent the widening "digital health divide", a term used to describe the disparity between older (and lower) versus younger (and higher) users of healthcare technology.

COMBATING AGEISM IN DIGITAL HEALTH

Colleagues in all healthcare disciplines should challenge ageism and embrace and support older adults' use of digital health. The modification of ageist beliefs and practices starts with raising our collective awareness. We can re-examine blind spots instilled by society and the medical model of aging, which emphasizes loss and dysfunction over wisdom and growth. This may decrease self-blame or defensiveness from singling out individual healthcare professionals for displays of ageism. Greater buy-in from healthcare professionals and training opportunities to build digital health competence could improve the provision of services to older patients. To promote digital inclusion, we must collaborate on improving access to health services and participation in transformational research. Below are concrete strategies for clinicians and researchers to promote equitable digital health practices with older patients.

Education and training

Educators play an important role in preparing the healthcare systems to provide quality and equitable digital health for older adults. The widely documented lack of formal education in geriatrics and digital health among healthcare professionals suggests that enhanced training is needed at all career stages. These knowledge gaps can be filled by the interdisciplinary field of gerontechnology, which specializes in matching digital health to the diverse needs of older adults. Gerontechnology curriculum on the appropriate, effective, and ethical use of digital health with older adults can be implemented throughout healthcare systems, such as onboarding programs, yearly compliance courses, and continuing education on digital health best practices. These topics can form the basis for core digital health competencies for healthcare providers across research, clinical practice, and at the organizational level. Research is needed to determine whether these educational interventions can lead to greater acceptance among healthcare professionals and increased use of digital health with older patients.

Clinical practice

Consistent with standards in geriatrics and general medicine, providing quality and equitable digital health services starts with a comprehensive biopsychosocial assessment. Clinicians should assess the multitude of factors that influence digital health readiness, such as preferences, access to technology, sociodemographics, health literacy, and impairments during routine medical visits. Older patients with low digital health readiness could be matched with individualized needs, such as technological support from a medical assistant or providing devices when available. Prior research has identified various evidence-based skills clinicians can use to teach older adults new digital health technology. These can include a combination of engaging caregivers, linking to personal relevance, allowing time for experimentation, and avoiding common pitfalls (e.g., speaking too loudly or slowly). We encourage clinicians to follow guidelines for delivering digital health interventions (e.g., National Council on Aging) with older patients and promoting digital inclusion in healthcare settings. Improving the quality of clinician-patient interactions using digital platforms may also lead to further downstream effects, such as reduced staff burnout, increased patient adherence, and greater efficiency of appointments. However, additional research is needed to confirm these healthcare outcomes and determine the most effective strategies for improving the uptake of digital health in routine practice, particularly with underserved older populations.

Inclusion in research studies

Increased representation of older adults is urgently needed across the planning, execution, and translation stages of digital health research. Older adults can participate as key stakeholders through various methods, such as patient advisory boards and community-engaged studios. Feedback from older adults is valuable for preventing poor design choices, refining digital health interventions, and increasing the likelihood of implementation into healthcare services. Research can increase representation by broadening eligibility criteria and modifying procedures that disproportionately exclude older adults (e.g., multiple comorbidities). This will generate more data on the potential to leverage digital health for multimodal assessments and treatments of comorbid conditions that become more common with aging. Modifications (e.g., large bold font), consultations (e.g., address privacy concerns), and support (e.g., caregiver involvement) can promote perceived ease of use and increase participation [. Study designs can use digital health to reduce the burden of participation (e.g., passive data collection) and compensate for cognitive or functional limitations (e.g., reminder systems). Including older adults as end-users will help break the cycle of digital health being developed for and by younger people.

DIGITAL HEALTH INITIATIVES

Current initiatives, such as BLINDED FOR REVIEW and BLINDED FOR REVIEW, demonstrate the ability of clinical research studies to address current barriers to using digital health with older patients.

BLINDED FOR REVIEW is a 9-week cognitive behavioral therapy program for insomnia tailored for older adults. The BLINDED FOR REVIEW program incorporates evidence-based modifications targeting older adults, such as changes to the user interface (e.g., increased text size) and instructional design principles in intervention delivery. Over 300 older adults were successfully recruited and enrolled for an internet-based efficacy trial of BLINDED FOR REVIEW. Concurrently, older adults with mild cognitive impairment were recruited from memory and aging clinics for a pilot study to determine the feasibility and preliminary efficacy of the same BLINDED FOR REVIEW intervention The intervention required a wrist-worn actigraph nighttime for 2 weeks at baseline and post-assessments. In-person recruitment for this population was critical for rigorous diagnostic purposes and determining feasibility for future trials. BLINDED FOR REVIEW and actigraph watches were found to be feasible and acceptable for this population. Study findings suggested refinements, such as providing technological support via phone and consistency in study-specific tasks.

BLINDED FOR REVIEW is a live video mind–body and walking program that teaches older adults how to manage chronic pain and early cognitive decline. BLINDED FOR REVIEW integrates several technologies for both clinical and research purposes, including live video (to deliver the intervention and assessments), a wrist-worn digital monitoring device (for real-time step count tracking and reinforcement of walking goals), and smartphone apps (to access skill recordings and log weekly homework). Research assistants are trained to assess participants' familiarity with technology (e.g., experience with Zoom, devices owned), identify individual preferences (e.g., text, email, or phone communication), and create individualized support plans (e.g., specific family members who can help). In qualitative exit interviews, participants reported that encouragement from study coordinators, scheduling learning sessions, and on-call technical support helped overcome initial intimidation with technology. BLINDED FOR REVIEW showed high feasibility, acceptability, and satisfaction when delivered virtually and with remote data collection. A subsequent remote efficacy trial is expected to increase the recruitment of a more diverse older population by budgeting for devices and wireless plans.

CALL TO ACTION

Digital health has reached a critical point. Advances in digital health allow for greater personalization, scalability, and sustainability of healthcare services, enabling a precision medicine approach to promote the health and well-being of diverse aging populations. Yet, older adults risk becoming marginalized from our increasingly digitized healthcare system. We believe that ageism among healthcare professionals, that older adults are unable or unwilling to use digital health, and not solely the ineptitude of older adults, has widened the digital health divide. The actionable strategies and initiatives in this article offer a roadmap for overcoming these ageist beliefs and practices in research, clinical practice, and training. By achieving digital health inclusion, we can increase access, provide preventative and comprehensive care, and decrease healthcare costs for older patients. A growing number of older adults recognize the potential of digital health, and it is time for healthcare professionals to join them.

Purpose

Philosophy and Spirituality: Finding Purpose in Later Life

Persistent population aging worldwide focuses on modifiable factors that can improve later life health. There is evidence that religiosity and spirituality are among such factors. Older people tend to have high rates of involvement in religious and/or spiritual endeavors, and it is possible that population aging will be associated with the increasing prevalence of religious and spiritual activity worldwide. Despite increasing research on religiosity, spirituality, and health among older persons, population aging worldwide suggests the need for a globally integrated approach. As a step toward this, we review a subset of the literature on the impact of religiosity and spirituality on health in later life. We find that much of this has looked at the relationship between religiosity/spirituality and longevity, and physical and mental health. Mechanisms include social support, health behaviors, stress, and psychosocial factors. We identify a number of gaps in current knowledge. Many previous studies have taken place in the U.S. and Europe. Much data is cross-sectional, limiting the ability to make causal inferences. Religiosity and spirituality can be difficult to define and distinguish, and the two concepts are often considered together, though, on balance, religiosity has received more attention than spirituality. The latter may, however, be equally important. Although there is evidence that religiosity is associated with longer life and better physical and mental health, these outcomes have been investigated separately rather than together, such as in measures of health expectancy. In conclusion, there is a need for a unified and nuanced approach to understanding how religiosity and spirituality impact health and longevity within the context of global aging, in particular, whether they result in a longer healthy life rather than just a longer life.

Conclusion

Eating healthy is very important. Not only for you to live longer but to keep you out of the doctor's office and be off medication which may cause other harm to your body. Follow all the information mentioned above, and you will get good results. You would also be able to see up to your fourth generation.

About the Author

Cindy Martin Nagel has worked in the health field for 20 years and has always been health conscious, even as a kid. She grew up with my mother, who always gave her fruit instead of candy or junk food for snacks.

She has a bachelor's degree in business administration with a concentration in healthcare and a master's degree in healthcare administration. In her twenties, she wrote a documentary that aired on TV about how to eat healthily and live longer. So, healthy habits have permanently been embedded in her soul.

About EV Publishing LLC

EV Publishing is an online publishing service that aims to provide affordable publishing services to independent authors and publishers. Our goal is to empower writers to bring their work to a larger audience while lowering the cost of publishing.

To contact EV Publishing :
Website: evpublishing.net
Email: evpublishingllc@gmail.com